Na
Newbie!

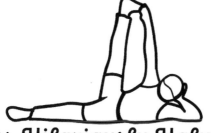

My *Hilariously Holy*
First Year Practicing Yoga

and a Simple Guide to
Getting You Started

by JIM DANT

© 2020

Published in the United States by Nurturing Faith, Macon, GA.
Nurturing Faith is a book imprint of Good Faith Media
(goodfaithmedia.org).
Library of Congress Cataloging-in-Publication Data is available.

ISBN: 978-1-63528-130-9

For Harper and Andrew
hoping they will inherit a more peaceful world

Acknowledgments

Every new adventure is undergirded by encouragement. My entry into the world of yoga was made easier by a handful of individuals who knew its benefits and knew I needed it. After expressing the teeniest of tiniest bit of interest in beginning the practice, Henry and Jane Watkins delivered a yoga mat to my office. I must admit that it sat in the corner for a while, but it was a necessary nudge. Liz Delaney has provided the sacred space of Greenville (SC) Yoga for me to learn and grow. Matt Rolin led the first class I attended after connecting with Greenville Yoga. He was extremely patient with all my questions, my nervous peeking, and my tight hamstrings—well, tight everything.

Ali Teeslink picked it up from there. Ali's classes at Greenville Yoga became (and remain) my regular time of practice. She has shared adjustment suggestions when absolutely necessary, but she has given me plenty of safe space to find myself in this practice.

I truly need to thank the whole staff and my fellow patrons at Greenville Yoga for being a community for me. I've practiced with almost all the teachers there and alongside people who have become either friends or sacred, familiar faces on the journey. Jenna Manning (church operations coordinator at First Baptist Greenville) has kept my overwhelmingly busy calendar clear enough to keep me committed. Between multiple meetings and writing and flying and speaking and counseling and a host of other things, she has given me the gift of managed time. Joy Yee has been a true friend. She has encouraged me and supported me as I've jumped off yet another cliff of interest.

They hardly know it, but the baristas at The Chocolate Moose at M. Judson Booksellers in Greenville and the owner/staff of M. Judson Booksellers have provided me with the space and caffeine necessary to complete this manuscript and share my yoga story. Who doesn't love a locally owned bookstore with a built-in coffee shop!

Finally, a shoutout to my daughters, who have each found their way to mindful practices—in one form or another—and have been wonderful examples to me.

To everyone who has helped me on this journey, namaste.

Contents

Foreword

It started with coins. Not just any coins—wheat pennies, buffalo nickels, and other unique pieces of metal from parts of the world that my six-year-old brain could not yet comprehend. I spent hours raking my hands through piles of shiny metal, examining images, dates, and other details (P for Philadelphia, D for Denver, etc.). I think back on the delight of finding that special piece, the thrill of popping that little coin in the cardboard cutout, and the satisfaction that another piece of the collection had been completed. Coin collecting was Dad's first "thing" I recall. "Dad's things" are what my sisters and I call his hobbies, passions, and pursuits, as we play phone tag amongst the three of us and joke, "Dad's on to his next thing!"

Around age eight the thing was hunting. I remember sitting on the floor in the garage of our Baxley, Georgia, ranch home (geography plays a certain role in determining the things), working to perfect the turkey call. It wasn't a loud guttural throat gobble disturbing neighbors multiple houses down. Instead, it required the use of a unique box instrument with the lid rubber-banded to the base, chalk drying the walls of the box. When rubbed together just the right way, the lid of the box replicates the perfect turkey call. I was actually pretty good at skeet shooting with the little .410-gauge shotgun my dad actually LET ME SHOOT at age eight! I have a horribly embarrassing picture of Dad and me decked out in camo gear, getting ready for a day of deer hunting on Grandma's property. (My adult self cringes at this disregard for ahimsa, the yoga practice of nonviolence. But let's be honest: neither of us was ever going to really shoot a sentient being—at least I wasn't.)

Around the same age the thing was piano. Dad was taking piano lessons, and I was too. For me the piano lessons went on for six years. For Dad, not quite as long, but this propelled me into a music journey that extended to marching band and concert band in high school, pep band in college, and Dad and I jamming on our ukuleles during my wedding reception.

While growing up in his home, I observed Dad jump into a number of things through the years, and I'm sure there were many more things during the years prior to my existence. I can recall him pursuing golf, running, biking, swimming, cooking, and guitar playing, just to name a few. I left my parents' home at age eighteen. For the past fifteen years I've been in my own space, exploring my own things. I no longer follow my dad's course, but clear my own. I appreciate he instilled in me the necessity of hobbies, passions, and pursuits outside of work. It's essential for community building, connection, and self-care. My own "things" have included local theatre, ukulele playing, Krav Maga, tarot reading, and yoga, just to name a few.

One connection I notice in each of "Dad's things" is the necessity of mindfulness and meditation. You have to practice mindfulness to sort through hundreds of coins, sit in the woods in complete silence, and play a piece of music. Running, biking, cooking all involve quiet time with the self. It makes sense that Dad would eventually gravitate to yoga.

Dad didn't initially tell me he was beginning a yoga practice; one of my sisters did. I called her to ask how her visit to Greenville went, and she said, "I went to yoga class with Dad. I think this is going to be his next thing." I was delighted to hear this, as I had established a yoga practice a couple years prior. Of course, in typical Dant fashion (if we get into something, we get ALL in), I immediately bought Dad a strap, blocks, bolster, all the necessary yoga props, to gift Dad for the next holiday. At a more core level, I could feel my inner child's excitement that Dad and I again had a thing to share.

While my sisters and I banter about Dad's things, I do acknowledge the minimization of passions in using the word "things." Dad sets a great example of modeling his passions as a way of life, and necessity for balance and self-care. I am looking forward to seeing how yoga is incorporated into Dad's lifestyle and how it continues to nourish him in mind, body, and spirit. This book, *Namaste, Newbie!*, provides a glimpse into Dad's first steps into his new thing. I hope it will inspire readers to find their own "things" to enhance their ways of living.

The light in me honors, reflects, and respects the light in each of you. Namaste, newbies.

Lauryn Dant

Introduction

I am not an authority on the practice of yoga. I am, in many ways, deciding to be the proverbial blind leading the blind. I am a beginner offering insight to other beginners. I am a novice sharing my embryonic experiences and pitifully sophomoric thoughts in order to get you past whatever anxieties and fears you hold with regard to yoga. Some may seem simple: What equipment do I need? How will I ever learn the poses? Will my body really do that? Other concerns may be deeper: Will this conflict with my faith? Do I have to be vegan? How will yoga affect my life?

I am making the assumption that my experience and subsequent thoughts will naturally address the mental and physical obstacles that have kept you from entering the yoga world, your local yoga studio, or your community center's yoga class. Some fellow novices will be astounded by the depth of my knowledge and commitment after having only practiced for one year. Longtime practitioners of yoga will probably smile and roll their eyes at my ignorance and naivete. Both reactions will be expressions of truth.

I want this book to be informative and fun. I want you to laugh *with* me and *at* me. I will transparently expose my worries, missteps, and fumbles so that you can either avoid them or fall fearlessly into them. I would suggest the latter.

I'll admit it: I want to entice you into a world—no, into a way of being in the world—that makes the world a better place for all of us.

Yoga and Doritos

Someone has to do it. I was paid to board an airplane, fly to California, and speak at a religious youth camp. I flew into San Francisco (my home away from home) and made my way to a beautiful retreat center nestled in a redwood forest just north of Santa Cruz. Like I said, someone has to do it.

Outside my teaching sessions, the youth retreatants were led in daily adventures that stretched their boundaries of life and personal comfort. The week's adventures included surfing lessons, a midnight hike through a state park forest, and a yoga session. I hopped on a van with the anxious teenagers and made my way to Ananda Yoga in Scotts Valley, California. Admittedly, I've always been somewhere between the sophomoric critic and the uppity expert when it comes to yoga. If the point is physical, I found myself making fun of downward dogs and happy babies as compared to the rigors of ironman training. If the point is spiritual, I am an ordained minister. I have stretched the limits of my personal spiritual practice through meditation, centering prayer, the Ignatian Exercises, certification as a spiritual director, multiple theological degrees—well, you get the picture.

We hopped off the van and stepped into Ananda Yoga of Scotts Valley. Yudhishthira Andrews (Doug) met us at the door. With a gentle spirit and a genuine smile, he welcomed us to the studio. He ushered us to the cubbies where we put our shoes, valuables, and other unnecessary personal belongings. He introduced us to Mary Nipper, our teacher. Mary gave us a brief overview of yoga practice and then settled us onto our mats. She guided us through an hour of breathing, poses, and intentions.

As we ended the final resting pose (she called it savasana), we were guided to a seated position, received a blessing, and shared responsively the final word—*namaste*. I thought to myself, "This is Doritos!" (And now for my first lengthy parenthetical diversion. You will find these throughout this book. They are indicative of the bouncy connections my brain makes when writing. I hope they aren't annoying. Feel free to skip all parenthetical statements. But if you do, you'll miss the fun stuff. So a moment of deep self-disclosure: Doritos are my drug of choice. If I eat one Dorito, I eat the whole bag. It matters not how large the bag happens to be. I know they are not the healthiest snack in the world, but I love them—every flavor: taco, nacho, cool ranch, sweet chili, etc. So naturally, I have sworn off Doritos. I might sneak off and eat a bag once a year, but I run by them in the grocery aisle. My life would be consumed with Doritos—and I would be thirty pounds heavier—if I ever allowed them pantry space in my home. Wow, it sure felt good to get that off my chest.) So that was my first thought: This is Doritos! This is too good. This could be addictive. But I don't need one more thing in my life—one more addiction in my life. Addictions cost time and money! I'll have to fit yoga practice into my schedule and yoga clothing, yoga books, yoga stuff (I've seen people toting mats and water bottles and blocks and all sorts of things), and yoga classes into my budget. I refuse to adopt one more hobby, passion, or addiction!

Five months later, in mid-December, I was five years into a large church pastorate. Our church boasts over 2,000 members; almost 100 people on payroll; 240,000 square feet of buildings and acres of campus. In addition to my day job, I was writing, traveling, speaking at conferences, teaching, playing bass guitar in an R&B funk band, training for triathlons, and doing all the other things humans tend to do (eating, sleeping, celebrating holidays, vacationing, spending time with family, going to movies, etc.). Life had sped up and filled up on me. My usually slow way of being—even in a fast-paced environment—had given way to the flow of contextual traffic. I began wondering what I could do to regain my slow, deliberate, intentional sense of self. My mind raced back (because that's the only speed it knew at the time) to the quiet savasana that ended my yoga session at Ananda Yoga of Scotts Valley.

We're all going to be invested in something (or addicted, if that's your perspective). Why not be addicted to or vested in something that benefits your whole self? I chose yoga. On Sunday, January 6, 2019, I drove to Greenville Yoga—just three blocks from my house. (Yep, I was part of that "New Year's resolution crowd." I'm sure a few people saw this awkward, middle-aged man and thought he wouldn't last past February.

What they didn't know was this wasn't about resolutions or fitness or diets. This was about reclaiming a life.) I wandered into the lobby where a posted sign proclaimed, "You belong here." I tentatively walked into a yin yoga class, laid my brand-new mat on the floor, laid my nervous body on the mat, and waited for class to begin. The journey started at 4:30 PM. I'm still on the path. Life is still full, but I'm moving slowly, intentionally, peacefully, gratefully, and happily. And as awkward as it felt at first, I now know I do belong.

Do I Really Have to Learn Sanskrit?

When I entered the world of yoga, I had no idea how complex this particular subculture's language would be. I had learned the language of many prior subcultures. I am part of the musical subculture and am fluent in the areas of theory, musical genre, instrumentation, and notation. I'm a runner, so I can talk all day about PRs, energy bars, and fartleks (I'll let you look it up). In the world of poker we constantly share information about ranges, tells, pot odds, and river rats. Like all other subcultures, yoga has a language all its own. It is an interesting combination—a meshing and mashing—of ancient Sanskrit and (in my case) southern English.

I stepped into my third class, was welcomed with a warm smile, and was told I would need a blanket, a strap, and a bolster. (For my first two classes, I had brought a mat. My "yoga daughter" told me I would need a mat. A church member had purchased a mat for me. I had a mat.) I had read an online description of this particular class prior to arriving. It was a restorative yoga class (yet again, more language). Restorative yoga is supposed to be among the easiest of all yoga practices. It involves no more than three poses or postures, all on the floor, with joints completely supported, and you relax for an hour. At check-in, I was told I needed a strap and bolster. My thoughts? "I'm not here for the sadomasochism class; I'm here for restorative." Being new, I kept my thoughts to myself and simply asked, "What is a strap and a bolster, and where do I get them?"

As you regularly attend classes, the language expands. Like a child processing their first auditory experience of words, you will hear phrases, process phrases, and attempt to connect phrases to immediate experience in order to ascertain meaning. The instructor says, "Come to a comfortable seated position and find balance on your sitz bones." Did she say *sit* bones or *sis* bones, or is it spelled *cis* bones, or did I even hear the word right? I rocked back and forth until the bones in my butt felt, well, balanced. I'm certain she didn't say *butt* bones. (It's sitz.)

After a few moments of quiet, guided breathing, she invites those who have an ujjayi breath

(I'm lost again) to engage that practice. From this static position, I was then instructed to move into child's pose, sphynx pose, seal (if I felt like it), downward dog, runner's lunge, airplane, warrior two, mountain pose, tree pose, forward fold, temple pose, and finally down to hands and knees. Before moving to our backs, we were invited to take a couple vinyasas if we wanted. Again, I thought to myself, "Is this a drink? Are they served in the lobby? Do they bring them to you?" The instructor continued her guidance with windshield wiper the knees, knees to chest, happy baby, and finally corpse pose. Yes, corpse pose. It's more often referred to by its Sanskrit name—savasana. In fact, all of these poses have Sanskrit names. Sometimes the instructor uses the Sanskrit. You either know it or you just take a few extra breaths and peek to see what everyone else is doing. If everyone is peeking, you're in trouble. In reality, the Sanskrit designations of these asanas (another Sanskrit term, which simply means "poses") are rarely used. English terminology is much more common, and it won't take you long to learn.

It is not just the language of asanas that I've learned in yoga. There are other terms that permeate this subculture's verbiage as well: forgiveness, patience, persistence, practice, gentleness, enough, rest, presence, honesty, generosity, nonviolence, contentment, and more. There are Sanskrit words for all of these concepts too. But knowing the Sanskrit isn't nearly as important as simply integrating the words into your life.

Kindergarten for Grownups

If you feel the least bit intimidated by yoga, allow me to put you at ease. Yoga is essentially kindergarten for grownups. I realize this is of little consolation to those of you who stood outside your kindergarten classroom clinging to your parents' knees, crying with reluctant heels dug in, refusing to enter the strange environment on that first day of school. That moment, however, is years behind you. You've either recovered from it or repressed it, so don't let it hinder you.

Upon entering the studio, we all have cubbies—those little shelves and cubicles where we stuffed our lunchboxes, jackets, hats, gloves, and sundry other items as preschool children. There have been cubbies in every yoga studio I've attended. During the yoga session, the items are either "watched over" by studio staff or the outside doors are locked until the yoga session has ended. I always leave my shoes, socks, mat strap, keys, telephone, and jacket in my cubby. I'm telling you, it's just like kindergarten minus the lunchbox! (I guess I could bring a lunch box, but that would be unnecessary.) So if you have any anxiety about where to put your stuff while you're practicing yoga, relax—they have cubbies!

Not only do we have cubbies, but we are also provided an assortment of toys at the yoga studio! Your yoga instructor will call them props, but I prefer to think of them as toys. There are straps (typically used to assist with stretches), bolsters (pillows used to sit on or place under various body parts for soft support I've actually seen these in two shapes: a large Vienna sausage or Spock's coffin from *Star Trek: The Wrath of Khan*, which looks like a flattened hot dog), blankets (which may be folded to simulate bolsters, used as padding for knees and other sensitive body parts that contact the floor or as a coverup for naptime—see next paragraph), and blocks (a little larger than a standard brick, these are used to provide support for joints when practicing particular poses. Some are made of foam and tend to be softer; I like these. Other blocks are made of cork or wood and tend to be harder; I don't like these. People often combine blocks and bolsters to create wonderful support systems for their back or legs. Just watch and learn. They are the Legos of the yoga studio.

Again, I digress). Congratulations! You have just read the longest and most convoluted sentence in this book!

In addition to cubbies and toys, we are also offered naptime during every yoga session. Depending on the type of yoga class you are attending, the length of your nap will differ. In a flow yoga class, postures are changed in coordination with your breath—every breath, every other breath, or after a certain number of breaths. At the end of the class, the instructor will guide you to lie still for your final posture—savasana. While savasana will be discussed more fully later, it is a final resting pose and usually lasts five to ten minutes. In yin yoga, each pose is held for about five minutes. If you can fully relax into these shapes, you can take ten to twelve naps an hour. (This ain't gonna happen—the poses call for a degree of concentration—but suggesting you can take ten to twelve naps provides a nice chronology of yoga types). In restorative yoga, you will be guided into three or four shapes in one hour. These shapes are all on the floor and completely supported. Yes, you may actually fall asleep during each of these postures— three long naptimes. Finally, in nidra yoga, you maintain one restful position for the entire session while being guided in a unique form of meditation. Nidra is often referred to as the sleep of yoga. Depending on your body's energy levels and needs, yoga truly provides not only an opportunity for the expending of energy but provides holistic rest as well—or, as I like to call it, naptime.

Cubbies, toys, and naptime create a kindergarten environment for adults. While these details may seem trivial to some, it is often the simplest concerns that cause us to avoid new adventures. The "not knowing"—with regard to process, equipment, and other seemingly obvious elements—can be a powerful deterrent. There's no need to stand at the door of the yoga studio clinging to your internal parent voice, crying with heels dug in. Step across the threshold and play.

Yoga I Have Yet to Experience

Yoga can be a quiet life. It is for me. Unlike being vegan, a cross-fitter, or a bagpipe player, there is no need to inform the world of your practice. (Okay, I'm not sure if bagpipe players talk about bagpipes all the time, but vegans and cross-fitters certainly do. No offense to my vegan and cross-fitter friends; it just is what it is.) The extent of my public announcements concerning my yoga life is limited to two yoga stickers on the back of my car, a yoga mat in the hatch of my car, and the fact that I invited a yoga teacher to attend our latest staff retreat so our whole staff could practice yoga in the mornings and evenings. (Okay, the staff probably thinks I'm no different from a vegan or a cross-fitter. But outside my immediate staff, I'm pretty quiet about my yoga life.)

A friend of mine recently discovered I was practicing yoga. She excitedly engaged me: "I practice yoga too! Do you want to attend a hot yoga class with me?" Being new to the yoga life and having limited knowledge of all forms of yoga, I asked her to tell me about hot yoga. She explained that it is just like regular yoga, but it is performed at a room temperature of 92–105 degrees Fahrenheit. This promotes profuse sweating and the cleansing of unwanted poisons and waste from your body. (She actually said all of this with a sense of excitement. I think she's a closet vegan and cross-fitter.) "So," she asked, "do you want to come?" I'm a man of few words. I simply responded, "No." And in the words of Forrest Gump, "That's all I have to say about that."

There are several yoga practices I have not tried. In addition to hot yoga, I have also avoided aerial yoga and paddleboard yoga. Aerial yoga—sometimes referred to as suspension yoga—utilizes straps or ropes (okay, it's a sling-like hammock made of very soft but durable material) suspended from the ceiling. The participant drapes their body in this suspended contraption, allowing their head, arms, and legs to hang out in different postures as gravity does its work. At its best it looks like Cirque du Soleil. At its worst it looks like elegant traction.

I've also not attempted paddleboard yoga. Don't get me wrong—I enjoy the water. I like fishing. I've been on a cruise. I've completed multiple triathlons—even an Ironman distance that required a 2.4-mile swim! Last year, I hopped on a surfboard for the first time and caught my first wave. Water is fine. I'm just not sure, however, I want to be floating mid-lake, attempting to keep my right leg wrapped around the back of my neck while balancing on my left leg on a paddleboard. (I can't do that on a mat in a yoga studio. I'm not even sure if that's a real posture. I was just making it up for effect. Apologies.)

Each of these practices—aerial and paddle-board yoga—takes the weight of my body off the security of the ground. I'm just not ready to do yoga in the air or on the water. I like the earth. Earth feels safe. (Several years ago, I completed a speaking engagement in rural Mississippi. That evening, I made my way to the small airport in Greenville, Mississippi. A prop plane with seating for eight was waiting to carry me and three other passengers to Tupelo, Mississippi, and then to our final destination in Atlanta, Georgia. Our luggage was loaded, we were boarded, but just before we left the gate, our pilot shut the engines down. He informed us a "warning light" was lit on the control panel and we could not take off until a mechanic checked and cleared the plane. We waited and waited. It was rural Mississippi. In about forty-five minutes, a 1965 Chevrolet Custom truck pulled onto the airfield. A gentleman stepped out of the cab of the truck, clad in overalls, hair disheveled, looking like he had been rudely awakened from a nap. He stepped into the cockpit area, looked at the light, walked to the back of the plane, and pushed the tail flap up and down. He came back to the cockpit and told our pilot, "It's your 'rear flap light' that's lit up. That usually indicates there's a problem with the rear flap, but it looks all right to me."

"Well," the pilot responded, "the light is still on, and it will not go off."

Ever knowledgeable and reassuring, the mechanic countered, "Well, it's kinda like that 'check engine' light on your car. It comes on all the time, but it don't mean anything." And he got in his truck and drove off.

We flew to Tupelo and on to Atlanta. Here's the deal. When my check engine light comes on and my car stalls or stops, I'm on the ground. I can pull to the side of the road. I don't need a check engine light coming on while I'm in an airplane, a few thousand feet in the air. I digress.) I don't need to do yoga in the air or on the water. I like the earth.

So, for now, I'm going to stick with yoga on the ground in a well-ventilated, comfortable, temperature-controlled setting. But that's just me. You do you.

I Have Always Liked Pigeons

Bird-watching is one of my many hobbies. I have a Peterson Guide to most regions of the United States and a couple for other countries. I used to obsessively check off each avian species on the day they were spotted. Today, it's less of an obsession, but a new sighting is always a reason for rejoicing. I like all birds. I'm not particularly partial to migratory anomalies in a region or the rare glimpse of a nocturnal bird of prey. Really, I like all birds. I even like pigeons. I could sit on the steps of St. Paul's Cathedral and sell pigeon food for two pence a bag (obscure reference to a song by the Sherman brothers featured in the 1964 motion picture *Mary Poppins*). I could have played Brenda Fricker's role in *Home Alone 2* (equally obscure reference to the bird lady in the 1992 Christmas comedy). Both of these cinematic characters were surrounded by pigeons, and that would be fine with me. I know the owners of belfries and statues and clean car windshields do not like them, but I think they are beautiful. The bird family Columbidae includes doves (the smaller) and pigeons (the larger). Their plumage can be dull and gray or quite translucent and ornamental. They are found worldwide—in the driest regions of the Sahara and in the cold polar regions of the Arctic and Antarctic. They are sturdy and strong and resourceful and relatively friendly—and, yes, they poop a lot. Many people hate pigeons, but I like them.

I've heard a lot of yoga friends complain about pigeons. Pigeon, however, has become one of my favorite asanas (poses). It didn't start that way. I'm not even sure how to describe pigeon to you. I can only tell you how it feels. When a yogi guides you into pigeon, it feels as if they are attempting to dislocate your hip, knee, and ankle all in one fell swoop. But once you get it and are able to relax into it, it's a great stretch!

There are several other asanas I enjoy: child's pose, thread the needle, melting heart, support-ed bridge, and cobbler's pose. I'm not sure how many asanas exist. I've heard mention of twelve basic poses; eighty-four poses if you adhere to the list of tenth-century yogi Goraksha Sataka; 8,400 variations of Sataka's poses (if you're a mere mortal); and 8,400,000 variations (if you are a completely self-actualized, enlightened, nirvana-dwelling entity. I'm not quite there yet). I'm a beginner, so the ones I have mentioned are relatively easy. As my first year progressed, I encountered more challenging poses (at least for me) than pigeon: warrior three, half-moon, and saddle to name a few. I've attended special workshops to help understand the techniques for some of these asanas. During these workshops, instructors—with your permission—will help move your body into achievable variations as you learn. There is never a reason to avoid the practice of yoga because you don't think you can achieve an asana. It's called *practice* for a reason. We all practice.

More importantly, however, the spiritual nature of yoga is not accomplished in one's ability to physically master a posture. Most of the value—as I have experienced it and understood it—is in what you notice while in a particular posture. What thoughts arise? Where are you tense or tight? How does breathing vary? Does the posture evoke happiness or anger or frustration? How are emotions felt and managed while in a particular pose? The physical exertion of yoga certainly benefits the body, but its potential for a deepened self-understanding and a broadened spiritual connection are the greater benefits. As Swami Kriyananda has written (*The Art and Science of Raja Yoga*), "[Yoga postures] were originated not by football coaches and P.E. teachers, but by great sages who recognized in certain postures the outward expressions of inward movements in the soul." (Wow, I just quoted a Swami! I must truly be on the path to enlightenment!)

Pigeon is my favorite pose. Savasana is everyone's favorite pose. At the end of each yoga session, we completely relax on our backs. Every muscle and joint are melted, weighted into our mat. Our eyes are closed. We rest. We are still. Savasana.

Savasana is commonly called the corpse pose. It is not only a pose that rests and honors our body after a workout, but it is a pose intended to prepare us for our deaths. Please don't think this morbid. Sleep serves the same purpose; it is a preparation for death. This reality is embedded in the poetic prayers of our children: *Now I lay me down to sleep. I pray the Lord my soul to keep. If I should die before I wake, I pray the Lord my soul to take.* It is an idea embraced by monks and mystics. When we sleep, we relinquish control of our lives. We are unaware.

We trust we will either awaken or be ushered to a new reality via death. Every time we close our eyes to sleep, we are practicing for our death. The same is true of savasana.

I wouldn't mind dying in a yoga studio. I would not want to wish hosting my death on the other students or the teacher or the owner. But they might handle it better than other people in other places. I'm pretty sure my fellow students and yogis would "get it." And I'm pretty certain I'm not the first to have entertained this thought. I can imagine being in savasana…breathing naturally…and then…in a moment…I exhale… my last…soft…breath. After everyone else rolls to their side, mindfully sits up, receives their blessing, and engages the response of namaste, someone will notice I am still in savasana. A student close to me will check my pulse. That same student will say, "He's dead." And I truly hope someone in the room reverently but confidently exclaims, "What a great way to go! I'm glad it was him and not me. But what a great way to go!"

Okay, that got a little morbid. I really wouldn't mind dying peacefully in savasana. But today I'm alive, and I choose to be a pigeon.

Don't Try This at Home

With all this talk of postures and pigeons, it's easy to allow the newbie anxieties to creep in. They are always lurking just at the edge of my mat. Several times I've been tempted to simply practice at home. Yoga video instruction is available on DVD at any bookstore or sporting goods store. If you don't want to purchase a DVD, there are complete routines provided online. Why in the world, I questioned, would I want to go to a studio and try this stuff in front of other, more accomplished yoga students?

Let me just be short and sweet. Don't try this at home. A home or private routine will eventually be part of any yoga student's practice, but early on, the instructor and the community are necessary. The yoga instructor is able to watch our early practice, affirm our progress, answer questions, keep us from pushing too far, provide alternative postures for the unique structure of our bodies, maintain an awareness of our personal injuries and other health-related issues, ensure balance in our practice, provide a spiritual dimension to the session, and hold a safe space for us. Rarely can these necessary elements be accomplished in a video lesson.

Beyond the role of the instructor, I have found the community to be necessary. I've gained much from the modeling, encouragement, common wobbling, and quiet presence of those who practice with me. Our presence in each class is truly a gift to ourselves and to each other.

So I'll keep this chapter short and sweet. Don't try this at home until you have a comfortable practice in the studio.

Namaste, Newbie!

I attended a kirtan class during my second month of yoga. This is a yoga practice I failed to mention a couple chapters ago, probably because it isn't as dangerous as aerial and paddleboard yoga—at least physically. Kirtan is a beautiful mix of hatha yoga (physical poses) and bhakti yoga (adoration for God). I'm using the word *God* here because that is how I name the object of my sacred affection. Everyone in the room will not use that language. We will discuss this at length later, but it is important to remember that yoga is a practice and not a religion unto itself. Prayer is a part of many faiths. Prayer is a practice, not a religion. People worship, perform acts of service, study sacred texts, and meditate in many faiths. Again, these are practices, not religions unto themselves. Kirtan is the devotional practice of yoga, which has the capacity to be as sacred as worship, as casual as simply enjoying the songs, and anything and everything in between. The participant is free to engage the practice at whatever level their personal faith or lack thereof desires.

Our kirtan class began with a traditional series of physical yoga poses. We then settled onto our mats—seated or lying down—and our leader led us in musical chants while he accompanied us on a harmonium. This may be one of the coolest instruments in the world. (I love music and musical instruments. I have spent way too much time and money in the world of musical instruments. As an elementary school student, I picked up a saxophone and it was my primary wind instrument into college. Of course, during concert season, someone had to play the bassoon. I was amazed by the quirky, giant stick, so I volunteered. In middle school I bought my first guitar—a Silvertone Acoustic from the Sears catalogue. That guitar began a long trek through a Yamaha, an Ovation, a Fender electric, a Gibson electric, three Dauphin classicals, a Kenny Hill Signature classical, and the pursuit of a classical guitar performance degree as a forty-five-year-old return-to-college student. There were a few more guitars purchased here and there. This is not the end. I was asked to learn bass guitar to accompany one song for one singer on one particular night. So of course I bought a Fender Precision bass and then a Fodera Monarch and then a Supro Short Scale bass and then a Zon fretless bass, and now I play bass in an R&B funk band. In the cracks along the way, I've taken piano lessons, learned to play harmonica, purchased and played three ukuleles, and, well, I think you get the picture. I've spent way too much money and time in the world of musical instruments—in some people's opinion, but not mine.) I want one of these harmoniums! It looks like an amalgamation of a pipe organ (typically two octaves of keys and seven stops), an accordion (the traditional instrument has a manual bellows and the sound is produced by air) and a suitcase (it folds into a suitcase-sized box with a handle). Okay, the first royalty check from this book goes into purchasing a harmonium. (Thanks for your donation.)

After we had postured and sang, the yogi invited us to sit in a circle. He asked, "What is the one thing you wish to gain from your practice of yoga?" His eyes glided around the circle, landed on me, and he said, "Let's start with you. Tell us your name and what you wish to gain from your yoga practice."

I'm usually slow to speak. I rarely open my mouth without a sense of intent. But in that moment, I spoke before thinking. I immediately responded, "Community. Family."

I couldn't believe these words had come out of my mouth. I immediately sputtered into a defensive and wordy explanation. I told the group that I was actually at this studio so I *would not* be known. I am the minister of a fairly large local congregation. We even host yoga classes at the church. I avoid these classes, however, because everyone knows me there. One of the things I love about the yoga studio is the pseudo-anonymity I enjoy. Very few people actually know who I am or what I do for a living, nor do they care. I can slip in the door, roll out my mat, close my eyes, practice, and leave without ever engaging a conversation. On other days I am free to chat with instructors and other participants—casually or at times more purposefully. But there are no expectations. No one needs or wants anything from me. I can talk or not talk, smile or not smile, greet everyone or greet no one. I can be wherever I want or need to be on a particular day, and everyone "gets it." Everyone lives with the same freedom. So, I'm not sure why I said I'm here for community and family.

The verbal diarrhea finally stopped flowing. I looked around the circle at everyone. They were looking at me. I saw no judgment in their eyes; I saw a lot of understanding. It seemed everyone knew what it was like to be part of communities, families, and gatherings that you truly loved, but that also held the capacity for exhaustion and expectation and dysfunction. They also knew what it was like to walk into the yoga studio—a place where you could just be, where you let others just be, and you chose to be together on the healthiest of terms.

My eyes followed the circle of everyone gathered there, finally falling on the yogi leading our class. He repeated my words, "Community and family." He stared at me—eye to eye—for what seemed like minutes, but I'm sure it was only seconds, and then he said, "Namaste. I see you."

Exactly How Many Muscles Are in the Anal Sphincter?

I was surprised to learn there are only two muscles that constitute the anal sphincter—the internal and the external sphincter muscles. The external is a relatively flat muscle that stays in constant contraction since it has no antagonistic muscle. (Biceps and triceps are antagonistic muscles. The contraction of one allows for the extension of the other.) The internal muscle is a smooth cylindrical tissue just inside the anal canal. These two muscles work together to prevent the leakage of solid waste, fluids, and gases from the rectum. They work—most of the time. The muscles are primarily involuntary—they work without you thinking about them. But they may be put under a greater or lesser degree of contraction if influenced by external stress or strain (squatting, bending, sneezing, etc.) or through intentional mental will—deciding to relax or contract the muscles.

I passed gas in yoga class. There is no other way to say it. (Well, there are other ways to say it, but they are a bit juvenile.) There is no way to ease into the subject. I just did it. It was not on purpose; who would do that? Okay, what fifty-something-year-old would do that? But as my recent research suggests, if certain external stresses or mental intentions are applied, the sphincters will release. I've thought of this often during yoga. There are several yoga poses that are just like cocking a gun for the anal sphincter: child's pose, happy baby (maybe that's why babies are so happy), forward fold, downward dog, temple. Each has a way of potentially adding a little strain to that area. My misfire, however, was not the result of these poses and their inherent stresses. Mine was the result of mental intentions. Our class had relaxed into savasana. Our instructor decided to make absolutely sure we were relaxed. She verbally guided us from the crown of our heads to the tip of our toes—inviting us to relax our head, neck, forehead, face, jaw, shoulders, arms, hands, fingers, chest, back, abdomen, pelvis, glutes, thighs, knees, calves, ankles, feet and toes. (Are you with me?) I relaxed everything, just as instructed. When savasana ended, she invited us to roll over on our sides and then mindfully make our way up into a seated position. I had intentionally relaxed everything. But when I sat up, I forgot to intentionally tighten everything. You know the rest of the story. If you relax every muscle in savasana, you better tighten back up before you sit up. I'm just saying.

Yes, I passed gas in yoga. It was not the silent kind either. It made some noise. Lots of noise. Loud noise. No one giggled. No one commented. No one looked around with suspicious or accusatory stares. It was one more reminder that people who practice yoga are in touch with their humanity. We don't mind our humanity showing. We appreciate the authenticity of our fellow humans. We can truly relax in our own skin because we are a community that affirms the beauty of our humanity.

Namaste is a combination of two Sanskrit words: *nama*—bow; *ste*—you. It literally means "I bow to you." It is most often understood to mean "I see you" or "I acknowledge you." *Hreste* is the Sanskrit word that means "I hear you." No one ended class on my special day with that word, but they could have—and it would have been okay.

Every Yogi Has
Their Own Voice

Jill is everyone's first-grade teacher and spiritual director. She delights as much in the verbal instruction and explanation as she does in the actual practice. This is a good thing. She is patient, intentional, and caring. There is no doubt about where she is leading you, what she wants you to experience, and the gentle provision of guarded space to get you there.

Lynn's voice embodies the serious business of hatha yoga. She excels in clarity. Her voice has an element of demand. If she told me to stick the big toe of my left foot into my right ear, I'd find a way to do it or die trying. It is not a harsh or coercive voice, but it cannot be ignored.

Ali is my regular yogi. She is a participatory meditative type. For easy postures, she stands obscurely at the back of the room and softly speaks instruction. For more difficult postures, she is on the mat at the front of the room, gently voicing and visually shaping options for each asana. When poses are held (particularly during yin practice), she is typically quiet. Sparse instruction may be given—reminding you to bring your mind back to the moment, relax the muscles in your forehead, or breathe. She has an inviting, permissive voice that sets me at ease.

Kimmie is everyone's best friend and sister. She is an incredibly delightful creature. If you weren't practicing with her, you'd want to be partying with her. Most yoga classes I attend employ background music that is meditative, New Age, or Eastern in sound. I've never attended one, but I've heard Kimmie has led classes to the likes of Beyoncé, Billy Idol, and Johnny Cash. (Okay, I haven't heard she's used Johnny Cash, but I can imagine it.) Kimmie's voice is challenging. She watches you and verbally pushes you to your edges. It's not her voice, however, that is most unique about her. It's her sound effects. When we're in a really good stretch, she often releases a wonderful sound. It is somewhere between a moan and a sigh, between ouch and preorgasmic. We usually get about three per session. I look forward to them.

Matt's yin class is filled almost every Sunday afternoon. We are wall to wall on our mats. He is the master of yoga-babble. This, in no way, is meant to be critical or insulting; it's just what is. When I'm in a room speaking, people accuse me of religio-babble. I'm constantly using ecclesiastic terms to speak about biblical, theological, and religious issues. And while people may get the gist of what I'm saying, for many it's just babble. Psychologists often engage in psycho-babble—descriptions of human behavior in academic and medical terms that can be generally understood but actually mean little to the lay listener. Matt is the master at telling us about the meridian lines that are separating our organs and lining up with lunar equinoxes that coincide with Chinese philosophical insights while stress is being held in the mandible because the farm where he was raised has a creek and it's a full moon outside. You get the picture. I kind of understand it. It certainly assures me he knows what he's doing. I'm still not certain I understand it all. Everyone else in the room seems to understand. I'll get there.

Liz. I'm not going to talk about Liz. She owns the studio and sets my membership fee rate. She has a perfect voice.

Here's what I need you and all my instructors to know. I love their voices. I love the different perspectives they bring to the mat. I delight in these voices. Each of their voices speaks to me, guides me, comforts me, challenges me, reassures me, and nurtures me in a different way. The voice in you may not hear them and respond to them in the same way I do. And that's all part of the miracle.

Holding Space for Human Vulnerability

You will be asked to assume postures in yoga that you would not feel comfortable doing in front of the family at Thanksgiving dinner. It just needs to be said. In a reclined cobbler's pose, you lie on your back and place the soles of your feet together (creating a diamond shape with your legs), opening your pelvic region. In downward dog, forward fold, and cat postures, you will press your rear end back and upward. In temple pose, you will squat like you are going potty in the woods during a long hike. (This is an assumption on my part. I've never been on a long hike in the woods and needed to go potty.) A variety of poses press the heart forward—and while many may think this to be of no consequence—it feels threatening to those who hunch to hide and guard their hearts. While in these postures, you will often be asked to close your eyes—yes, close your eyes in a room full of people you may barely know. The instructor will almost always add, "Only close your eyes if it feels safe."

There is an inherent vulnerability in the practice of yoga. But here is what I want you to know: Our instructors hold this space for us. Yes, I read the news. I know there are persons in this world intent on taking advantage of people's vulnerability. And yes, there are a few yogis who have breached the ethics of this sacred space. But every instructor I have known has held a safe space for those who engage the practice of yoga. They stand over us in our vulnerability to ensure no one takes advantage of us.

At our studio, this happens in some very practical ways. The outside doors are locked when practice begins, and the interior doors are closed. We are encouraged to close our eyes or softly hood them to keep our attention inward and not on others in the room. We are encouraged to hold sacred each other's dignity. We are told no one will ever take pictures of us without our express permission. (Apparently, a few yogis over the years were so enamored with the beauty of a room full of people in silent savasana that they took pictures. This was considered trespassing a person's vulnerability and is not allowed.) Our instructor stands or sits near us during savasana—symbolically and practically guarding us and watching over us as we rest.

How many safe spaces really exist in the world anymore? How many places are you able to open your heart and your body to the heavens and know that you will not be harmed physically or spiritually? How many places can you exercise mind, body, and soul without looking over your shoulder, being aware of your surroundings, and assessing every human that moves into close proximity? A female friend of mine recently told me the one thing she longs to do but cannot is take a walk alone in her neighborhood at night and look at the stars. Sadly, she said it will never happen.

I've spent a lifetime looking for safe space. I have never been physically assaulted or physically abused, but I have lived life in successive contexts of anxiety, uncertainty, and manipulation. My biological mother lived through a cycle of bad relationships. As a very young child, I found myself navigating who was sober, who was mad, who could be trusted in any moment, and who could not. I was eventually taken from this home and spent a period of time with extended family and in foster care. Again, at a young age I found myself assessing people and rooms and motives. I was adopted while in elementary school. This provided a stable home but, nonetheless, a new environment that required learning and adjustment. My adoptive parents divorced during my last year of middle school. Subsequent marriages forced a continued pattern of assessment and navigation in my life. And then there was the church—my faith family. While the church will always have my undying affection and commitment, there have been those within the church who used their authority to manipulate thought and used fear to manipulate decisions. The positive aspects of having lived through this personal saga are that I can read a room and read people pretty quickly. It made me a really good poker player. The negative result? I have lived a life filled with trust issues.

So here's the deal: I cannot guarantee your yoga studio or class will be a completely safe space—humans are humans. I have had the wonderful experience of practicing with a group of yogis who intentionally work to ensure the studio is a safe and sacred space. My body, my thoughts, and my faith are respected and guarded when I am in the room. If at any moment you sense you are not respected and guarded during your practice, leave that studio, but don't leave yoga. Find another place to practice and another yogi with whom to practice. Don't relinquish your well-being to someone else's depravity.

And finally, be part of creating and maintaining a safe space for others. Even those of us who practice have a responsibility to treat those who gather with us with deep respect. Keep your gaze inward. Give people space to safely be alone in a crowded room. Dream of a world where a woman can walk alone at night and gaze at the stars without having to glance over her shoulder—and at least make it so in the yoga class.

There Is Only One Mirror at Our Studio

There is only one mirror in the practice area of our studio. If you visit the studio, it will take you a while to find it. In my travels, I've been to other studios that have mirrors affixed to every wall. I find it tempting in these studios to stare at the mirror. I'm constantly checking to see if my back is straight, if my leg is lifted high enough, if my chin is parallel to the earth, if my feet are hip distance apart, and, well, you get the picture. For me, the more mirrors, the more self-judgment. Our studio only has one mirror in the practice area. It is the mirror within.

I have come to value the practice of noticing. External mirrors on a wall entice me to critique what each moment looks like. Noticing—the internal mirror—guides me toward integrating what I'm doing with what I'm feeling. It is less concerned with what I look like and more concerned with who I am.

I do not need an external mirror to tell me I can twist much easier than I can balance.

Asanas that require my body to bend and wrap and contort are typically easier for me than those that require a degree of equilibrium and steadiness. The practice of noticing allows me to see this reality reflected in my life. Twisting is easy for me; balance is harder. I can accommodate and adjust to almost any situation or person easier than I can stand in a place of balance. I can find a hundred ways to contort my time, resources, and opinions in order to accommodate what I think others need. This often disrupts the balance in my life.

Our bodies often reflect the nature of our lives. We live our lives in our bodies, so the tension, rest, flexibility, and balance (or lack thereof) we hold in our souls are naturally expressed in our postures. Early in my practice, I asked my instructor, "Do I have balance problems because I'm a guy?" She wisely responded, "You struggle with balance because you are you."

The internal mirror of yoga will always be more valuable than the reflective glass some studios hang on their walls.

No Judgment—
It Is Your Practice

She was in my second yoga class. I see her regularly now. She slid into the studio, unrolled her mat next to mine, laid on her back, closed her eyes, and never said a word. She also never followed instructions. Never. If we were seated, she was standing up. If we were in downward dog, she was in child pose. If we were lying down, she was seated. If we were in warrior two, she was in happy baby. I know I'm supposed to stay within myself, stay on my own mat, pay attention to my own practice, and not critique the practice of others. But she was never in sync with the rest of the class. She just did her own thing! I see her regularly now. Nothing has changed. She still does her own thing! (Noticing others is truly an early aspect of the yoga experience. The longer I practice and the more inward my focus becomes, the less I notice those around me. As one of my instructors is fond of saying, "Close your eyes if it feels safe. If that does not feel safe, keep them softly hooded. Keep your focus inward. There is nothing to see here.")

I'm a minister by trade—a member of the clergy, a preacher, a Baptist preacher no less. I have found corporate faith expression to be an interesting phenomenon. Allow me to oversimplify the history of religion for you: A long, long time ago, someone had a religious experience. In some form or fashion, they perceived the presence and/or power of God. Over the course of time—days, weeks, months, or years—they met other people who had perceived the power and presence of God in a similar fashion. For some it was in a sunrise, others in meditation, others in the sweaty act of service, others in a song, and others in an enlightened thought. The perceived experience of God and the connection with others who had the same experience were positive aspects of faith. The prior provided individual encouragement and the latter a sense of community. Where this all falls apart is when these groups of similar experience began to write it down, call it doctrine, and demand everyone else have the same experience. Are you still with me? And if anyone didn't have the same experience as the group—well, you know, they are destined for hell, utter despair, destruction, and/or the annihilation of the soul. (It's amazing the

58

eternal punishments we can conjure to impose upon people who are not like us.)

I'm a member of the clergy, a preacher, a Baptist preacher no less. But I have adopted and lived and worked with a perspective that has enriched my life, enriched my faith, and allowed me to learn from and love all people. It is simply this: When I am tempted to judge, I choose to wonder. I open myself to learning about other people's lives, faith practices, spiritual experiences, or lack thereof. Wonder allows me to feel at home in any synagogue, church, mosque, prayer circle, temple, home, or personal conversation. Wonder has taught me how similar we all are in our longing for the sacred, for community, for silence, for stimulation, for peace, for love, and for relief. Wonder allows me to celebrate our distinctiveness. Our differences are our greatest points of interest, our edges for learning, and the elements that provide our world with diversity. (I have a friend who delights in saying, "We would be completely bored if there were only one type of bird, tree, flower, or animal in the world, and yet we want every person in the world to be just like us. It makes no sense.) Yes, I have had an experience of the power and presence of God. And yes, I gather with people whose past and present experiences are similar to mine. But no, I do not condemn those who experience and express faith differently. I don't even condemn those who have no need for faith or faith expression. I wonder, I listen, and I learn from their experience. What a farce to believe that an infinite and invisible God can be limited or monopolized by any individual or any religion. How much more sacred and respectful it is to believe that the mystery of an infinite God is best expressed through an infinite number of experiences, perspectives, beliefs, and doubts.

I have been intrigued to learn that in the last two years, more people joined yoga studios than churches in the United States. I think I know at least one reason: no judgment. It's your practice. Whether you are down-dogging while I'm child-posing or you are following the teachings of Jesus or Buddha or no one's teachings at all, you are welcome.

That's Not Christian, Is It?

Sigh. Do I really have to write this chapter? This is like a plumber working on his own pipes. It's like a painter coming home to paint his own house. Do I really have to address the sacred validity of the practice of yoga? This is supposedly my area of expertise (although *expertise* might be an overstatement). I could write a book on the integration of yogic practices and religious faith; many others have. I, however, am going to keep this brief, experiential, and non-argumentative. (At least I am going to try.)

Yoga is not a religion; yoga is a spiritual discipline. Feel free to compare yoga to prayer or fasting or worship or generosity or the study of sacred texts. Almost every religious faith engages these practices, yet they are distinct religions. Yoga is one more faith practice that—like prayer, fasting, or worship—can provide a path to self-discovery and a greater connection to God. It can also be practiced with no religious basis or intent. This is also true of other spiritual practices. One does not need to be religious or even believe in God to study sacred texts, fast, or be generous. Yoga is not a religion; it is a practice.

I regularly see fellow church members in my yoga classes. I regularly see persons of other Christian denominations and other faiths in my yoga classes. I have friends who attend yoga and claim no faith. Our church hosts yoga classes throughout the week. Many other churches and faith institutions host yoga classes. The people I see in these classes are some of the kindest, most graceful, loving, generous people I know.

On the other hand, if someone sees the Greenville Yoga sticker on my car or hears me mention yoga in a sermon or sees me reading a book about yoga, I inevitably receive an article via mail or email reminding me that yoga is an evil, satanic cult. One such article was accompanied by a note that stated, "I know you are a minister *and you know the Bible*, but be careful that Satan doesn't lure you away from the church with this New Age thinking and you end up in hell." It was unsigned.

Okay, maybe I'll be a little argumentative. *I know you are a minister* and you know the Bible. First, you do realize the Christian Bible is an Asian, North African document? The translation of this book into English and it being absconded by Western Europeans has nearly depleted the sacred text of its original geographic ethos. The Bible emerged from the Middle East (that's Asia) and Egypt (that's Africa). Jesus was Asian. Jesus spent a portion of his formative childhood in Egypt (North Africa). The Apostle Paul's travels were intended to spread an Asian religious perspective throughout a world dominated by the European gods of Greece and Rome. The Bible is an Eastern religious text, not a Western religious text. Our reading of the Bible should at least allow for—if not demand—attention to its connection to the Eastern understanding of words, phrases, and practices. When you read the Bible and encounter words like *meditation, light, gate, breath of life, heart, vine, river,* or *tree,* you should be willing to explore the significance of these terms in Eastern culture rather than simply relegating them to our Western definitions and biases.

But be careful that Satan doesn't lure you away from the church with this New Age thinking. Second, yoga is not New Age; it's old age. The practice of yoga and yogic philosophy predates Christianity. And so it shouldn't surprise us that we see facets of yoga practice and philosophy in the life of Jesus: going into the mountains or wilderness alone, lying down in the bow of a boat during a storm, and ultimately the intrinsic gaze maintained during his crucifixion. While postured and dying on the cross, Jesus maintained a present awareness that spoke his personal sense of forsakenness, sought forgiveness for others, desired care for his mother, acknowledged personal thirst, and retained the self-control to "give up his own ghost." I could go on and on and on, but instead I challenge you to read the stories of the Bible and sift the words of the icons of the faith. You will find them immersed in the practice and language of yoga.

And you end up in hell. Finally, I do not believe in a personified Satan or the eternal damnation of any human soul in a place called hell. (Again, another book for another day.) But if your god sends people to hell because they sit in a room together, establish healthy community, spend time in prayer, take care of their bodies, honestly search their own souls, and depart to live kinder, gentler lives, you might want to shop around for another god. And as far as Satan goes, I've seen a lot more of him at church than I have the yoga studio. (And you know how much I love the church.)

I've listened intently to a few Christians who have found yoga offensive. In my opinion—and it's only my opinion—their concerns are seeded in their own faith insecurities. I can't imagine a person who has truly relaxed into the grace and love of God being threatened by the practice of yoga. There is nothing in the practice of yoga that has diminished my Christian faith. Challenged it? Yes. Deepened it? Yes. Enhanced it? Yes. Diminished or assaulted it? No.

Understanding Yoga Fashion

I would like to say a word about yoga fashion. I'm certain there are those with whom I share a studio who would argue I have no credibility in discussing this issue. In the hallways and darkened corners of the studio, they have probably whispered about me, "Have you noticed he wears the exact same shirt to every yoga class?"

For the last two decades, I have been an avid participant in the Leukemia Lymphoma Society's Team in Training program. I have run numerous marathons, cycled in centuries, and competed in triathlons in order to raise money and awareness for those suffering with blood cancers and those working to find a cure. No one in my family has suffered from this type of cancer. That is part of the reason I participate. I am grateful for the health we have enjoyed, and as an act of thanksgiving, I run, bike, and swim for those who are battling these diseases. Motivations, however, are often mixed. The selfish side of me enjoys seeing the world. Team in Training jets athletes across the United States and around the globe to participate in competitive events. We raise designated amounts of money to participate. The bulk of the money goes to patient care and research. A portion of the money affords our travel. It's a wonderful program.

For each event as a Team in Training participant, I am given a purple Team in Training singlet to wear on race day. They all look alike. The savvy eye will notice some difference in graphic, but the variance is so slight that the average onlooker—who only sees them separately, on subsequent days, for about an hour, in a dimly lit yoga studio, while their eyes are closed most of the time—will think it's the same shirt. I have a dozen of these tank tops. I rotate them. I don't wear the same shirt every day. I just wear the same type shirt every day. (This is also true of my wardrobe when I am away from the yoga studio. I wear solid-colored, button-down oxfords every day: white, blue, pink, or lavender. It just makes life simpler. Recently I was visiting my four-year-old granddaughter. She was sitting in my lap, and I was reading her a book. All of a sudden, she forcefully slaps her palm onto the open page, looks up at me, and says, "Stop!" I stopped reading and asked, "What's wrong?" She responded, "Pop, do you wear the same shirt every day?" Her parents burst into laughter. They would all fit in perfectly at the yoga studio.)

In recent weeks, I've added a few graphic t-shirts to my yoga wardrobe. But on most days, you will still see me rocking the purple tank tops associated with Team in Training.

I mention all this to reassure you: Don't fret over your yoga outfit. There is no doubt that yoga clothing has become a fashion trend. There are tights and tanks of every color, design, and pattern. It is the preferred shopping garb and travel wear for a lot of people. But you don't have to worry about being fashionable while practicing yoga. Wear what is comfortable to you and what feels good against your skin. Make sure you have a good range of movement in the clothing and that it isn't binding or restrictive. Spend hundreds on the most fashionable tights, or just wear your old sweatpants. And if you still can't decide what to wear, call me. I've got a few Team in Training tank tops I'll loan you.

You Think You're Incognito

I dare say most Americans think of yoga as simply one more form of exercise. In our fitness-crazed nation, the masses have typically associated yoga with health clubs and gyms. Yoga's purpose is too often relegated to attaining some measure of flexibility, strength, and balance. Yoga, however, is historically a multifaceted practice. Its primary purpose is to provide stillness and balance in the individual and in the world. Hatha yoga is the physical practice of yoga—the practice with which most Westerners are familiar. Other expressions of yoga are jnana (study and wisdom), bhakti (practice of devotion), and karma (practice of surrender that often expresses itself in good works).

I practice hatha yoga five days a week at my local studio. But I also practice other forms of yoga in my life. These forms of yoga typically take place within the context of my chosen faith expression. As stated earlier, yoga enhances my particular faith identity. It gives new language to what I have experienced on my faith journey. It does not contradict or detract from my faith.

Quite the opposite. It brings a discipline to my life that makes fuller engagement in my faith possible. Jnana yoga is the practice of study. I am practicing jnana yoga each time I read, meditate, dissect, ponder, wrestle with, and exegete a sacred text. This practice of study allows me to also take seriously other writings and lectures. I am able to listen, be present, and attempt to understand how another human being sees, experiences, and responds to the sacredness, beauty, and suffering they find in life.

I practice bhakti yoga in my worship, private prayers, and meditation. These are my forms of devotion to the higher power I call God. This certainly happens in the context of my particular faith tradition where hymns, prayers, litanies, and sermons are offered. My yoga studio is also church for me. What gathering could be more reflective of the mystery of an unseen God than a gathering of people who engage God with different names, different images, different practices, and different experiences? All of us come together to reflect the many facets of the jewel, the treasure, that is our God. We are humbly admitting no one has a monopoly on God, but are instead willing to quietly be in the presence of what we consider holy.

Since I spend a lot of time in my mind and a good deal of time on my mat, karma yoga is a practice I must intentionally engage. I would consider it my weak point. Karma yoga is the practice of doing good work in the world. In the walls of the church, we would call it ministry or service. Yes, I perform many acts of service in my role as a minister: visit the sick, sit with the lonely, provide financial assistance to those who lack, and more. But I daily do these things from a vocational position or station in life. By virtue of my office, I am expected to do these things, paid to do these things, recognized for doing these things, and held accountable if I neglect these things. This is good and necessary. But in my personal practice of karma, I want a greater purity. I want my service to be a gift. I do not want to be paid or recognized. My yoga family affords me the opportunity to practice karma.

During the Lenten season (forty days of prayerful preparation before Easter) of 2019, a Period Packing Party was advertised on my yoga studio website. It was posted as a karma yoga opportunity. I had been a member of the studio for about four months. I was barely familiar with karma yoga and had no idea what a Period Packing Party was. I called the studio to ask the basic questions. First question: What is a Period Packing Party? Answer: Volunteers gather to put an assortment of feminine hygiene products in Ziploc bags and then deliver them to homeless shelters, prisons, schools, and other institutions where less advantaged women can have free and easy access to these necessary products. Second question: Is it okay for a guy to participate in this party? Answer: Of course! We need all the help we can get!

A week later, on a Sunday afternoon, I showed up. I had rid myself of the Sunday morning robe and clerical vestments. Donned with faded jeans and a gray hoodie, I walked into a room full of strangers—an anonymous giver, a practitioner of karma yoga. I was assigned a table with four other volunteers, and we began neatly stuffing tampons and pads and liners into the provided bags. The other volunteers at my table were friends. They chattered delightfully throughout the process. I listened. I smiled, nodded, or laughed when appropriate. Otherwise, I simply enjoyed my time of clandestine service. The table talk subsided into a momentary silence. We fell into the quiet rhythm of counting, stuffing, zipping, and stacking. It was in this lull of chatter that the lady next to me leaned over and whispered, "You think you're incognito, but we all know who you are. Thank you for what you and your church do for our community." I looked up, and the whole table was smiling at me. So much for the unrecognized purity of karma yoga.

Here's what I have learned about yoga and life: I'll never get each yoga asana perfect. In fact, I'm not sure there is a perfect yoga pose. All of our bodies are different, and each pose has a bit of variance when coupled with the beauty of our unique physicality. My study, devotion, and service are not going to be perfect either. I'm not even sure what perfect would look like! My practice of yoga will always be marked by my humanity. I love it when I see this in others. I have learned to appreciate this beautiful stroke of humanity in myself. I don't have to be perfect. In all aspects of my life and faith, I'm just practicing.

Jungle Medicine

I was ordained to the ministry in November 1983. I was barely twenty-two years old and was a year away from finishing college. I had not been to seminary. I had never studied theology. But hey, that's the way we Baptists do it. In many religious traditions, an ordinand (candidate for ordination) must complete a graduate degree in seminary, be mentored by a senior minister, and pass exams in orthodoxy (proper beliefs) and orthopraxy (proper faith practices) before being ordained and assigned a ministry position. Baptists, however, believe in the autonomy of every local church. The local church is not governed by a larger denominational structure. In other words, each church—large or small—can practice faith in the manner they feel led. As a result, many Baptist churches—particularly smaller ones—will choose to ordain and employ ministers who have not received a seminary education but have displayed some level of connection with the divine and the ability to communicate it. The individual church ordains the minister, and that is all the credentials they need. I was ordained in November 1983 and was barely twenty-two years old.

If you are cringing, it gets worse—or better, depending on your perspective. I had actually been preaching since I was in seventh grade. After a tumultuous childhood riddled with multiple divorces and a stint in foster care, I was officially adopted, in third grade, by a Baptist family in southeastern, rural Arkansas. Prior to my adoption, I had experienced faith as a Roman Catholic. I was completely enamored with Scripture, stained-glass windows, robes, incense, priestly vestments, and all things spiritual. I truly had an innate desire and drive toward the beauty and depth of the faith. As a child, I memorized Bible verses with the same passion with which many of my friends collected baseball cards. I loved the mystery of God and the practice of the church. My new life in the Baptist church was much different, but it was still my avenue of interest and meaning.

In seventh grade I was baptized into the membership of Northside Baptist Church in Eudora, Arkansas. After my baptism, I told my minister that I had always wanted to be a priest when I grew up, but now I wanted to be a

Baptist minister. (Be careful what you wish for.) With a huge smile on his face, he told me I would be preaching the next Sunday evening! (In rural Baptist life, when you feel "called to preach," the congregation assumes you have been blessed with this ability, and they expect you to preach—now—right now.) I still have the notes from my first sermon. It was seventeen points long and lasted five minutes. (There was very little illustrative material. But this makes sense—how much life has a seventh-grader actually lived?) I was hugged and hand-shook and congratulated on a job well done. I was then scheduled to preach once a month, to the small crowd of maybe thirty people, until I moved from that town. So by the time I was twenty-two, I had accumulated a degree of preaching experience. And while this may seem dangerous or ridiculous to some, you cannot imagine the opportunity it gave me to study, learn, struggle, and explore my faith. I, in essence, practiced jungle medicine for this brief period of time. (For those unfamiliar with the term, *jungle medicine* refers to the practice of medicine in a context of high need by a person who has limited knowledge or skill but is the best available.) I knew enough about the Bible to offer some help, comfort, and challenge to those in need. But in all honesty, I was not ready to serve a congregation as their pastor. Personally, psychologically, spiritually, and professionally, I needed the formative years of seminary and the shared wisdom of mentors, both of which I later received.

Years later, I found myself serving as a minister in South Georgia. I had graduated from college and two seminaries. I had served under a competent senior minister in a highly respected metropolitan church. I had submitted my personal human psyche to therapeutic counseling and formal spiritual direction. I was trained and ready to preach and pastor. One afternoon, a gentleman walked into my office and requested formal spiritual direction. During his prior residence in Atlanta, he had employed a spiritual director to give guidance to his life. I informed him that while I had also enjoyed the experience of spiritual direction, I had never been trained or certified in the work of spiritual direction. He pushed aside my lack of credentials, informed me there was no certified spiritual director in our county or the surrounding counties, told me he sensed

I was innately skilled at the practice, and asked me to be his spiritual director. I agreed—jungle medicine. (Just a few years later, I took a sabbatical and received my training and certification in the field. I eventually became certified in group spiritual direction, Ignatian Retreat direction, and I now teach in a certifying program. But, the fact remains, I was exercising the gift before I was officially trained. This seems to be the pattern of my life.)

All that said (and it was probably far more than you wanted to know), I had been practicing yoga for five months when I again made my way to the San Francisco Bay area of California. (I spend about six weeks each year in San Francisco. It is truly home away from home.) I had been invited to lead a spiritual retreat at a campground about seventy miles south of San Francisco. Upon arrival, I looked at the retreat schedule and saw a yoga class scheduled for Saturday evening. I could not have been more excited. I had already dreaded missing my yoga classes at home. I had established a pattern of practice that included flow on Mondays and Wednesdays, yin on Fridays and Sundays, and either restorative or nidra thrown in one day a week. The retreat began on Saturday morning. I led a morning session and then an evening session. After the evening session, I hustled to my room to retrieve my mat (yes, I carry my mat when I travel, just in case) and returned to the conference hall for yoga. About thirty other retreatants had gathered with towels or blankets, and we all stood there and stood there and stood there. The yoga instructor had not shown up. We were informed there had been a miscommunication and there would be no yoga session. The crowd was about to disperse when a friend of mine in the group said, "Jim, you take yoga. Could you lead the session?"

Here is how quickly my mind worked: "If I lead an hour yin session, the first few minutes can be breathing and relaxing, the last five minutes would be savasana, and that leaves fifty minutes to fill. If each pose lasts five minutes, I only need ten poses to fill the time. These are all beginners, so all poses can be on the floor. I have to make sure each pose has a counter pose for balance. I can do this." I felt a surge of confidence. I had been a jungle preacher and a jungle spiritual director. I truly can do this. But there was also some trepidation. The only risk in the prior situations—pastoring and spiritual direction—was the eternal damnation of someone's soul. In yoga, however, there are muscles, joints, preexisting injuries, and real physical consequences to consider! (No, I do not believe in the eternal damnation of any human soul. I do believe, however, in arthritis, knee and hip replacements, and tissue-related problems. There were real risks involved!)

I told everyone to lay their blankets and towels on the floor and to find a comfortable seated position. I explained to them I was not a yoga instructor, but I would be happy to have them join me as I practiced yin for an hour. I explained yin to them—a relaxed practice, holding poses for about five minutes each, never pushing too far into a stretch but just far enough to maintain our attention and always backing off if tension turned to pain. I told them not do anything that moved beyond mild discomfort. And if I asked them to do anything that felt painful, raise a hand and I would assist them in finding another posture.

We began on our backs. I guided them through preparatory breaths, windshield wipers to loosen the lower back with legs dropping to the right and then the left for five minutes each. We followed this simple twist with banana pose, reclining pigeon, and reclining pigeon twist. We then went to our front bodies to provide some counter poses. I instructed them to simply rest their heads on their hands if this was enough for their lower backs or move into sphynx pose.

After demonstrating each pose, I would stand and walk around the room. It was amazing to see participants from the teaching perspective. I could see people tightening shoulders and jaws and foreheads, so I would give gentle reminders to relax these areas. I noticed a few overly aggressive individuals shaking with tension and would remind them to pull in their navel to reduce tension on their lower back or breathe into the area of tension or back off the stretch if it felt like too much. In essence, I found myself mimicking the words and instructions of those who guided me in yoga, in much the same way I had followed the paths and verbal patterns of preachers and spiritual directors. We ended the session by pushing back into child's pose, and then we shifted to our backs for transitional knees to chest and then savasana.

When the time for savasana had ended, I invited the group to gently come back into physical awareness, gently move fingers and toes, roll over onto their sides for a moment, with eyes closed mindfully push themselves up into a comfortable seated position, place their hands at prayer in front of their heart center, and bow their heads to their hearts. I offered a short blessing for them and thanked them for sharing my practice with me. I spoke the parting word, *namaste* (no one said this back to me because it was outside their experience and I had not instructed them to do so), and told them the session had ended. We all opened our eyes. Some eyes were wet with tears. Others were smiling and stretching. Others began chatting with their neighbors. Almost everyone in the room expressed some form of gratitude to me, told me the practice was exactly what they needed, and a few wanted to talk about how to begin a practice of their own.

I find great joy in sharing things that bring me joy. I am a teacher by nature and find it easy to convey knowledge and experience. I had not begun my yoga practice with the intention of teaching. In fact, just the opposite. I wanted this practice to be "for me," without the responsibility of sharing and leading and teaching—those practices that already permeate other areas of my life and vocation. But I'm a teacher. As my first class trickled out of the conference room that evening, I decided I would pursue yoga teacher training at some point in my journey. Not because I want to teach a series of classes or own a yoga studio, but because that hour of guiding opened the door to all I did not know. It made me want to deepen my personal practice. And, of course, in the future if there is ever a group of people who want to practice—need to practice—and the scheduled teacher cannot make it, I want to be properly prepared.

They Don't Shoot Horses in Yoga

I love humor, but I'm not particularly fond of jokes. One joke, however, that has been stuck in my mind for years bears telling here. I'll keep it brief since I really don't like jokes.

A gentleman was riding his horse along a country road. A young man in a sports car sped by the rider and startled the horse. The startled horse lost its footing on the shoulder and tumbled into a deep ditch, where both horse and rider were severely injured. The horse had obviously broken a leg in multiple places. The rider had broken both legs and an arm and had suffered multiple lacerations. In a matter of moments, a gentleman pulls up in an old farm truck. He sees the horse and rider in the ditch. He pulls over and gets out of his truck to assess the situation. After looking at the horse first, he quietly walks back to his truck, gets a rifle from the rear window gun rack, and shoots the suffering animal. He then walks to the rider and asks, "Are you okay?" The gentleman looks up and responds, "I'm feeling wonderful. Thank you."

I had surgery just weeks after my yoga journey began. I had been suffering with an inguinal hernia for almost two years. My relationship with this hernia was getting harder and harder to endure, so I decided it was time to separate. Of course, this procedure required cutting and meshing and sewing and more recovery time than any human wants to accommodate. I had attended yoga long enough to know: 1) My practice is my practice, and I do not have to push myself into a shape that is painful; 2) I can inform the instructor of any "pains or problems," and they will help me with adjustments; and 3) there are special classes naturally oriented toward persons with pain or injury.

But here's the deal. We (okay, at least I) only want to be at yoga when we are at our best. Who wants to show up to yoga, or work, or life when they are their worst or weakest? Who wants to lie flat on their back or their belly in a room full of people holding warrior postures? I couldn't imagine hobbling into the yoga room, putting my mat on the floor, lying still for an hour while people practiced around me, accepting a helping hand to get up, and then leaving to await the next weak workout! But that's exactly what I did.

Two days after surgery, I made my way to an evening yoga nidra class. As previously stated, yoga nidra has often been called the "sleep of yoga." In nidra, we lie down and find one comfortable position. Participants remain in this position while the leader takes them through a guided meditation. It's challenging for the inner life, but easy-greasy on hernia stitches. Two days later, I was at a restorative yoga class. Again, as previously described, in restorative yoga, we lie on our mats for an hour and are guided into three postures. In each posture, props are used to fully support all joints. The purpose of restorative yoga is to find rest for the body and mind. While I regularly attend restorative yoga once a week, in my postoperative condition I was reintroduced to the practice as a wonderful context for healing.

Three days later, I hobbled into a class called Yoga for EveryBODY. I winced my way into the room, looked around and saw people in wheelchairs, people wearing various leg braces, people many years my senior, people restricted by other injuries or inabilities—but they were all people who showed up for yoga. In this class, we move through a series of postures, but we either remain seated in a chair or on the floor for the entire practice. If there are any postures that our bodies are unable to manage, the instructor comes to us and helps us find the right form for our condition. And yes, just seven days after surgery, I went to a full-on flow yoga class—and laid on my mat for an hour. My breath came and went with the synchronized breath of the class. I moved as my body was able—recalling postures from the Yoga for Every-BODY class. I kept going back—day after day and week after week—until I had forgotten the surgery had ever occurred.

What pushed me back into the studio so quickly after surgery? Part of my impetus was the guarding of ritual. Yoga had become a part of the fabric of my life. I attended particular classes on particular days of the week. The schedule was carved onto my calendar, carved into the physical expectations of my body, carved into my head and heart. I had come to depend on these moments of silence and movement and meditation and breath offered in this safe sanctuary—not the way an addict depends upon a drug of choice, but the way a body depends upon sleep or food or air. It was a part of the sacred movement of my life.

I was also drawn to the floor by a sense of community. We do not talk during a yoga session. I infrequently talk to anyone before or after a yoga session. But I missed them—those I knew by name and those I knew only by face. I missed the instructors. I imagined they missed me. I wanted them to know I was okay. I wanted them to "be with me" in the recovery.

I found my way to yoga when I believed I was at my worst and my weakest. What did I learn? There was nothing bad or weak about where I was in life—it was just where I was. Yoga is about being in the here and now no matter what the here and now happens to be. My community welcomed me back to the room and the floor—because they don't shoot horses in yoga.

Don't Forget to Breathe

Breathing is an essential part of yoga; it is possibly *the* essential part of yoga. Numerous books have been written about the intricate relationship of the breath with our mental, spiritual, emotional, and physical health. Rather than attempt to explain something I do not completely understand, allow me to share with you a few comments about breathing I have overheard in yoga classes (and a few other places). I trust these snippets of truth will convince you to look deeper into your own breathing practices.

If all you do today is lie there, breathe, and pay attention to your breath, you will have practiced yoga. Yoga is not ultimately about achieving a particular physical posture; it is about being attentive to the whole self. This attentiveness often begins, ends, and is encompassed by an attentiveness to our breath. It is the cool feel of breath entering our body and the warmer sensation in our nostrils and throats as we exhale. It is the extending of the diaphragm, the widening of the side-ribs, and the sensation of air in the back of our lungs. It is being attentive.

You should feel some tension in your outer hip. Breathe into your hip, and as you exhale, feel the discomfort leave the body along with your breath. The first time an instructor told me to "breathe into my hip, shoulder, calf" (feel free to insert any body part other than lung), I just quietly chuckled. The first time I tried it, I teared up like a needy man who had just experienced a miracle. Consciously breathing into and toward our pain allows us to exhale the pain and relax the once-strained tissues.

Don't forget to breathe. There are moments—while holding certain postures—that holding the breath seems to help. I do it (and I assume others do it) without thinking. For me, it's when I'm trying to balance. I unconsciously hold my breath. I need to be reminded to breathe. Breathing is necessary for living. (Duh.) And breathing during difficult times, stressful times, and times when it's hard to maintain balance helps us live more fully. And speaking of "holding" our breath…

Breathing reminds you to live generously. We take a breath, enjoy the breath, let go of the breath, and then trust—we trust—another breath will be there for us. This was another moment I almost started crying during a yoga session! I, like many, live my life in accumulation mode. Worried that there will not be enough (you name it: money, food, friendships, etc.), I hold to what I have. Yes, I live a fairly generous life, but I'm always aware of where my comfortable boundaries lie. I only release a certain degree of my resources, time, and energy. In many ways this is healthy, but in other ways—at its worst—it fosters worry. But to hear an instructor say "Take a deep breath in; take in a little bit more; hold it; now, release everything" reminds me not to hold too tightly to anything. Everything can be taken in, enjoyed, and completely released. The next thing I need will be provided.

Your breath is a reflection of your state of being. I pondered this statement for a long while, and I concluded it makes perfect sense. I draw in a deep and quick breath when I'm in awe. I sigh when I'm discouraged or disappointed. The pace of my breath—slow or fast—can indicate the level of my stress, anxiety, fear, calmness, and a host of other feelings.

Breath is the presence of the divine in us and among us. Most of the above quotes contained new information for this newbie. When a California instructor spoke these words over our seated, cross-legged bodies, she was preaching a sermon with which I am quite familiar. It is true. Breath and wind have been prominent images and indicators of divine presence in the literature and thought of many faiths. It is certainly true of my faith tradition. In Hebrew, *ruah* is literally translated "wind" or "breath." But of its 389 appearances in the Hebrew scriptures (Old Testament to Christians), over one third of the time it is a reference to God. In the New Testament, *pneuma* literally means "breath" but is most often translated "spirit" or "soul." In almost every Christian biblical lexicon, its first definition is "the third person of the triune God—the Holy Spirit." Countless biblical references could be cited illustrating the equating of God with wind and breath.

In the ancient creation stories, it is God's breath that brings life to humanity. Politically and religiously, a lot of energy is expended by a lot of conservative Christians arguing that life begins at conception. And while the Bible poetically implies God is involved in the formation, growth, and shaping of each child in the womb, a biblical literalist would have to concede the clear statement of life's beginnings as it is recorded in Genesis 2:7: "Then the LORD God formed man from the dust of the ground, breathed the breath of life into his nostrils; and the man became a living being." Life, and our attachment to the divine, is a result of breath.

So much more could be said, but I'll leave you with this wonderful thought from the ponderings of my spiritual cousins in Judaism: Some rabbinic scholars have suggested the personal name of God—Yahweh—is simply the sound of a breath—inhale, Yah; exhale, weh. When Moses asked God to tell him his name (Exod 3:13–15), God simply sighed; he took a breath in and let it go. The most respectful of Jewish persons will not speak this name of God. Many have translated the word to mean "I am who I am." I would like to think the name of God is simply a breath. If this is true, the first word we speak when we are born is the name of the divine. The last sound that crosses our lips before our death is the name of the divine. My California instructor was right: *Breath is the presence of the divine in us and among us.*

Don't forget to breathe.

You Might Cry

It was a Friday morning yin class. We were on our mats, on our backs, and had been guided into a side twist: "on an inhale pull knees to chest, on an exhale let your knees drop to the floor on the right, spread your arms like a T, tuck your shoulders under, open up your chest, hold, relax, and breathe." I was thinking about nothing in particular. I was relaxing physical areas that felt tense. I was breathing into spaces that felt strained. I was gently pushing my muscles and tendons and ligaments to an edge of sensation without pushing too far. I was lying still with absolutely nothing on my mind outside the sensations in my own body—and then I felt a tear trickle down the side of my face. And then another. And another. I found myself lying on a mat in the middle of a yoga studio crying.

Rather than worry what anyone else thought (I assumed they had their eyes closed) or try to stop the flow of tears, I just let them go. I began to wonder. (Because that's what I do.) What was I holding in? What about this posture generated tears? I surveyed my body and realized the dominant sensation for me was the openness of my chest. As instructed, I had opened my chest, tucked my shoulders, and spread my arms. Just thinking about this openness made the tears flow harder. Once focused on this part of my body, thoughts slowly surfaced with regard to people I was avoiding. In recent weeks, I had experienced some tense moments and conversations with two particular friends. At least for the time being, I had consciously and subconsciously walked different hallways and followed alternate schedules to guard myself from confrontation. I assumed we would find our way toward reconciliation and under-standing, but it didn't seem possible right now. The chest—the heart—that I had just opened on the mat had been closed for almost a week, concaved and guarded from people I truly loved. And when it opened, I cried.

Months later, I listened as one of our studio's yogis taught a class on forgiveness: "Our issues are in the tissues," she said. She went on to explain, "When we hold resentments, they settle into our bodies." I do not claim to completely under-stand this or to be able to explain it. There are a multitude of psychologists, physiologists, and yogis who have researched and written about the psychosomatic nature of our pains. Google an article or two if you need to understand it better. My point is simply this: You might cry. It is your practice, and you may do whatever you want, but I would suggest you let the tears flow—and wonder.

Is It Silly I Have Stopped Killing Bugs?

As previously mentioned, many students of yoga embrace the practice as part of their external beauty and fitness regimen. That's fine. No judgment. I have no stone in my hand, and I've never seen a stone in the hands of other yogis. This view of yoga, however, is relatively new and almost exclusively Western. I have found the deeper I dig into the philosophy of yoga, the more meaningful my physical practice becomes.

In the earliest days of my practice, I regularly brought my life to the yoga floor. When I laid down and my back felt the increasingly familiar "all natural, non-Amazon-harvested-tree rubber mat," my mind immediately began to race. I could conjure every past moment I regretted and every future challenge that garnered my worry and hope. I turned a corner in my practice the day I learned to take my mat into the world. Rather than focusing on my past or my future, I lived exclusively on my mat for sixty to ninety minutes.

The thoughts that kept me in the moment during each session were the five yamas (restraints) and five niyamas (observances) of yoga. These disciplines are found in ancient Indian texts that date prior to 400 CE. Volumes upon volumes have been written with regard to their origins, interpretations, and applications. I have no need to share an exhaustive history lesson or sermon with you. But allow me to quickly list the principles for you and tell you how I first incorporated them into my yoga practice and life.

The five yamas or restraints of yoga are:

- Non-violence (Ahimsa)
- Non-lying (Satya)
- Non-stealing (Asteya)
- Non-excess (Brahmacharya)
- Non-possessiveness (aparigraha)

The five niyamas or observances of yoga are:

- Cleanliness (Saucha)
- Contentment (Santosha)
- Self-discipline (Tapas)
- Self-knowledge (Svadhyaya)
- Surrender (Ishvara Pranidhana)

In recent months, I have spent more than a few hours studying these disciplines. However, before I ever read the history and origins of these principles, before I ever compared these principles to commandments from other sacred texts, before I ever studied scholarly interpretations and religious applications of these principles, I simply memorized them and then repeated one—just one—each time I laid on my mat.

I often arrive for yoga classes ten minutes prior to class. I unroll my mat and lie down for a few minutes of quiet. And now, rather than rush back through my past or scamper ahead into my uncertain future, I choose one yama or niyama and repeat it over and over again. When I leave that particular yoga session, I take that word into my day. I have found it interprets itself. Regardless of which principle I choose and mentally chant during the session, there always seems to be obvious application when I leave.

At a studio in California, my practicing neighbor screamed and fled her mat during a yoga session. A spider had crawled onto her mat, stopped at the corner, and seemed to be doing some cat-cow movements (a very common transitional asana—look it up on YouTube). I positioned my blanket in front of the little arachnid, coaxed him to crawl on, and took him outside. Nonviolence.

Months before, twelve of us had mats unrolled on an outdoor deck. It was a beautiful autumn evening in the North Carolina mountains. The stars were plenteous and light years above us. A single porchlight shown much closer—just a few feet away. It was the porchlight that drew the bugs. I was holding a plank pose when the palmetto bug (a fancy Southern term for a huge flying cockroach) landed on my mat just next to my left hand. I slowly dropped my knees, steadied myself, picked up a block, and beat the hell out of him. This was before I was introduced to the yamas and niyamas. I assume you see the difference.

The yamas and niyamas guide my daily decisions, actions, and attitudes. My familiarity with these disciplines has caused me to be graceful in arenas far beyond the insect kingdom. Regularly repeating these ten ideas—with no interpretation attached—has given me the strength and insight to wisely deal with a multitude of difficult moments in my life. I've stopped killing bugs. But I've also stopped killing time, killing dreams, killing personalities, and killing my own sense of self. And that's just nonviolence! Every yama and niyama has had deep effects on my life and the lives of those around me.

All Yoga Students Are Not Vegetarians

Ahimsa—the practice of nonviolence—is the first of the yamas. Like all sacred ideals, ahimsa has been interpreted and exercised in many different ways. For some it is limited to our treatment of fellow humans. This treatment not only forbids the physical violence we might inflict upon our fellow humans, but may also be interpreted to include the many other forms of mental, psychological, emotional, and spiritual violence we seem determined to deal out.

For others, as mentioned in the previous chapter, the practice of nonviolence extends to all of the earth's creatures. This is often seen in the eating habits of those who practice yoga. Many yogis and yoga students choose to be vegetarian and avoid the slaughter of animals for the purposes of nutrition. (I've actually read about a few yogis who will not even kill vegetation for nutritional sustenance. Instead, they claim to be able to feed themselves through breathing. They have so developed and evolved their yogic practice that they draw all the nutrition and energy their body needs from simply breathing. They are called breatharians. I'll not explain the practice further, but one published breatharian has stated that in his life, physical food is not necessary, but optional. "Oh, I can do that," I thought. "I'll breathe all my meals from now on. But once or twice a day, I'll opt to eat something." Sorry. I couldn't resist. I'm not critical, but I am a bit skeptical. But live and let live.)

Recently, I went to lunch with a fellow yoga student. I ordered a blackened salmon salad. She ordered the same without the salmon. She was visibly taken aback that I requested meat on my salad. She had assumed I was vegetarian because of my yoga practice. I told her I had experimented with being pescatarian once, but I kept finding myself with chicken, lamb, beef, and pork in my mouth. She was not amused. I asked if she enjoyed being vegetarian, and she quickly informed me she was vegan, not vegetarian. She went on to explain that vegetarians will allow themselves to eat some products from an animal, such as milk and eggs. Vegans, however, refuse to ingest animals or animal products. She walked me through a typical day in her diet, and I found myself immediately thrown into confusion.

"Wait," I said. "You are vegan, but you just recalled having milk on your cereal for breakfast. That doesn't make sense. Is this almond milk or some other plant-based milk?"

"No," she responded, "I'm lacto-vegan. I allow myself to drink milk for the calcium and vitamin benefits, but I am vegan in all other aspects of my diet."

After a moment of thought and a resulting epiphany, I gleefully looked at my friend and exclaimed, "This is it! This is the day! This is the moment that begins my vegan journey! I am a vegan!"

With the expression of an evangelist who had just won her first religious convert, she looked at me with wide eyes and responded, "Really?"

"Yes!" I asserted, "I am a lacto, fisho, beefo, porko, lambo, chickeno vegan! I can do this!"

She was not impressed.

I am not a vegetarian or a vegan or a pescatarian or a breatharian. I eat a moderate, balanced diet, and I try not to eat immediately before a yoga session. This all may change one day, but it is where I am right now.

Sometimes You Just Know

After my first yoga practice, I sent the owner of Greenville Yoga a note. After my first month of yoga practice, I sent the owner of Greenville Yoga another note. Here are the notes:

January 7, 2019

Good morning, Liz.

My name is Jim Dant. I am the senior minister at First Baptist Church here in Greenville. But...a different kind of Baptist. :-) I'm also a certified spiritual director, group spiritual director and Ignatian Retreat director. All that said...

This past summer, I found myself in an Ananda Yoga Gathering in San Jose California. I was leading a retreat there, and the hosts had planned a yoga session as part of the schedule. Put simply, it was one of the most refreshing, prayerful, life-generating hours of my life (and I've been in a lot of worship services). It made me realize "I" need some free/life-giving/ relaxed space in my life. I decided then I wanted/needed to incorporate yoga into the fabric of my life. But being the deliberate decision-maker I am, I held it for several months. The interest and desire did not fade, so I decided to start the new year with a yoga class. I attended yin yoga yesterday with Matt. First, he was a very welcoming and attentive guide. Second, it seemed to be a perfect class for a beginner like me. I plan to attend the 12:30 class today—mindful flow with Ali—and see how that feels and fits.

So I just wanted to introduce myself and thank you for providing such a "sacred space." I think it's going to be the perfect spot for this chapter of my journey.

Peace,
Jim

February 1, 2019

Hi Liz,

I promise I'm not trying to be a pen pal. I do, however, want to give you an update on my first month at Greenville Yoga.

I'm the type person who can step on a path and quickly determine if it will be a lifelong journey or a fleeting interest. The first time I went running, I knew—lifelong journey. The first time I refinished a piece of furniture? Fleeting interest. I picked up a guitar—lifelong journey. I played a round of golf—fleeting interest. I stepped into Greenville Yoga—lifelong journey.

I've attended four classes a week with Ali, Matt, and Pete. Each has been a wonderful guide in the early steps of this journey. I've begun reading a breadth of literature with regard to the history, philosophy, and practice of yoga. I wish I had come to this place earlier in my life, but I'm comfortable affirming we find our way to the right place in the right time. This is the next natural chapter in my personal pilgrimage.

All that said (and again, I promise I won't inundate you with emails), thank you for providing such a sacred, welcoming space. I truly look forward to pulling into that parking lot and spending time there.

Peace,
Jim

Sometimes you just know. It is certainly that way with me. As I stated in the second note, I've engaged a multitude of activities in my half-century of life. I've typically known from day one whether the momentary fancy would become part of the fabric of my life. There are many activities that have entertained me (adrenalin junkie) for the moment, but only a few that have sustained me for a lifetime: running, music, coin collecting (okay, I realize this seems far from an adrenalin junkie's activity of choice, but I can still remember as a child sifting through my change and finding a wheatback penny among the newer, shinier copper cents. It was a thrill. I guess you had to be there.), writing (I had a poem published in *Highlights Magazine* when I was nine years old. My work and my name were in print! I received a ten-dollar check in the mail! Adrenalin!), poker (another subject for another book on another day), and biblical studies. These passions have shaped my schedule, my relationships, and my life for years. I knew from day one that yoga would be added to this list. In fact, with the publication of this book, yoga has woven together all the passions of my life. It is a spiritual and physical activity (like biblical study and running), typically practiced to music (guitar), that I have written about (writing) in order to sell books and receive coins (coin collecting). But rather than taking the coins to the poker table, I'm gambling on the fact that these written words will encourage you to find your way to a yoga class. I can guarantee you a regular yoga practice will beautifully weave together the frazzled threads of your existence into a wonderful tapestry of life.

I haven't emailed Liz in a long time. Now I regularly pass her in the lobby of Greenville Yoga.

When she is not engaged in conversation, I make sure to thank her for the gift of this sacred space and her sharing of this sacred practice. If she is in a conversation with one of the other grateful souls, I try to catch her eye and smile. She knows. I know. God knows. And now you know. I hope to see you in class soon. Namaste, newbie.

Afterword

If you've just read Jim's book, he has painted such a delightful picture of what it's like to step into a yoga practice. He covered some of the most important topics, the deepest questions, and the hilarious moments that may occur. If he has inspired you to dip your toe in the water of yoga, then you will be forever in debt to Jim. (Just kidding. I had to add a little aside and humor in here too!)

Honestly, trying yoga may be the best thing you can do for yourself, your family, and your loved ones. At first you may resist this crazy practice, and the stillness may even irritate you, but I encourage you to keep going! As a newbie, here are some things you may want to think about and look for as you dip your toe in so eventually you can delve into the depths.

How to begin? First, search for yoga studios in your area. Do this by asking friends or asking around the community. View studio websites and see which one has the right feel for what you want. Want a workout? Look for the photos of sweaty, fit people in tight clothes. Want stress and anxiety reduction? Look for websites that create that feeling somehow—calm faces, images of lotus flowers and candles. Then think about your schedule. What is an easy time slot for you? What works best for your schedule? Don't worry about the names of the classes; instead, go to the ones that fit your timeframe. Start with once a week, and just see what you think. Try a few different studios and teachers. You will know the ones that resonate clearly with what you need and want in your life.

Once you have found a studio and a set of teachers you love, keep coming back (and read this part after you've been practicing yoga for a while). Somewhere along the way during your exploration of yoga, you may hit a bump. One day you are taking class and a teacher says one thing, or your body just relaxes in a whole new way and you may begin to cry. You may start to feel uncomfortable in your own skin. You may decide yoga just isn't for you. Here's the thing: Yoga isn't always shiny unicorns and rainbows. Yoga sometimes allows us to see the un-shiny parts of ourselves. The beauty of seeing your "stuff" is that you learn to accept it, to process it in a whole new way, and to let go. When you hit those bumps, I invite you to keep showing up. Keep practicing. Keep breathing. The only way out of the discomfort is through.

I was a part-time yogi for years. I started this journey in the mid-nineties in Los Angeles, a time when yoga was bursting forth in the United States. But it wasn't until I met my beloved teacher that yoga became a weekly habit and something I loved. Five years into dabbling in various yoga poses, classes, videos, and studios, I met my teacher, Max Strom. That very first class with him, I felt something completely different. We were in savasana. As I lay there, everything felt right. My mind got still and quiet. My mind wasn't already in the car and checking off my to-do list. My body felt lighter, almost nonexistent. I wasn't hungry or thirsty. And I felt, dare I say, relaxed! At the time I was as anxious as anxious could be. I was a wee bit controlling and a perfectionist. For those ten minutes all of that went away. I was content. I knew then that I had to keep coming back to learn from this man. I went once a week for a few months and then twice a week and then three times a week and then eventually five days per week.

I found that content feeling could last longer and longer, and it began to thread into my daily life. I became a recovering perfectionist. Life didn't quite feel like a pressure keg anymore. I learned to breathe and to relax my hold on everything. Eventually, I left Los Angeles, but the practice stayed with me. As Jim said, yoga didn't *replace* faith for me; it *restored* my faith. I went from tunnel vision of the things I needed to control (the mundane, daily things) to a wider lens that allowed me the see the beauty, the bigger picture. I could let go and trust my faith again. Yoga brought me home.

My hope for you is that if you are yoga curious, start right where you are. Don't worry; no one is looking at you! At the very least, your body will thank you for it (goodbye little aches and pains). At the most, it might change your life in the best way possible. There is no right or wrong on this path. Simply show up and breathe!

When looking for a studio, it may take time to find the one you like best. Here are things I looked for as a student and what we used to create a studio imbued with heart and meaning.

- Location: Is it easy for you to get there and park?
- Times: Are class times convenient for your life and schedule?
- Pricing: Are prices fair for the area? Is there some kind of sliding scale or discount? Should you fall in love with this, make sure it is sustainable for your budget as well.
- Intention: What are you seeking in your yoga? There are many reasons to start yoga: physical health, mental well-being, stress relief. Figure out what you are looking for and start there. None of it is wrong. I started yoga to lose weight, but something changed along the way.
- Studio: Is it clean and quiet? Is it about distraction or moving your attention in? As a side note, many of us studio owners use Buddhas or Indian statues as decoration. This is not meant to convert you to any religion or philosophy. Many of our statues came from TJ Maxx (not a very sacred shopping spot). But what they do show is a quiet smile and a serene face. These statues are often nothing more than a pleasing decoration. Do not let them offend you.

Instead, look at the smile of the Buddha and see if you can find that same smile.

- Teachers: Do they ask about your day, injuries, anything you need? Do they walk around and guide class or just practice yoga in front of you? Do they focus on achieving poses or alleviating stress and finding ease?

- Students: Is there a wide range of students in class (age, shape, gender)? Do people smile and say hi when they see you?

- You: How does it feel when you walk in the door? How do you feel during and after class? Do you want to keep coming back?

Liz Delaney, E-RYT, RPYT, YACEP
Owner, Greenville Yoga
Greenville, South Carolina